Eat How You Want to Feel
Guaranteed Best Way to Lose Weight, Get Healthy
& Feel Your Personal Best Ever!

By Robert Kintigh

Copyright

Forward

I have enjoyed this short book, and I am pleased to present to you a alternate life style in health and wellness. This book is dedicated tom the rollercoaster dieters who have struggled and fought to grind off a pound here and there. This book is for the person who just wants their clothes to feel comfortable and fit the way they would like.

I have been there myself, but along the way I played so many sports that my health always came back to a good place but only after I used great discipline.

Your weight is not all your fault, but you do have control over it all. The will to believe in this is powerful and so this little book is that big nudge you need to step back and take a new look at what it is you really want.

I am all kinds of failure too and I see you and hear you. I support you and get you. Your weight and health are not where it needs to be, but it is all right. It is going to be all right. Afterall, why can't you feel and look your best. Quit dieting and start succeeding in the lifestyle you have always wanted.

Be yo9ur biggest cheerleader and envelop yourself in the possibility that you can be your best. The true secret is that a healthy lifestyle starts with your mind. Get your mind in line and everything else should always follow. Quit with the toxic feelings, thoughts and people in your life. Purify the thoughts that have led to you being unhealthy.

Here is to you the struggling person as we look at a new idea of who you are and want to be……

Table of Contents

Introduction
Time to Change Lives

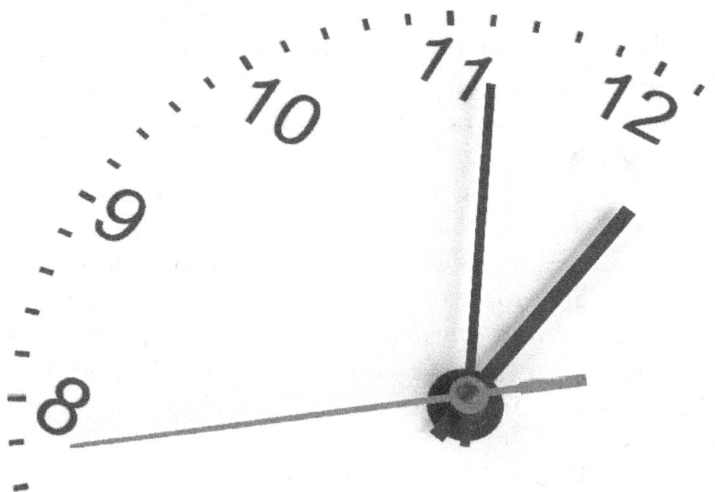

STOP! Everyone is tired of hearing about the salad you ate for lunch today. No, I am not being rude to you but, I am trying to break some very bad habits and obsessions that you might just have. There are two people in this world in my opinion that want to be healthy. There are the ones who always talk about it and those who just make it happen and do it every day without the talk. You are in one category or the other.

This is an interesting way to start a book on health and wellness but, the truth be told someone must shut you down, and get you out of your old routines and habits. Your friends and family just sit there and listen like they care, but they have heard this a hundred times and do not want to upset you. I on the other hand want to sincerely help you, and continuing the cycle you have been in for a long time helps no one.

If health and wellness is going to be in your near future then you will have to change many things in your life, get you moving some and eat how you want to feel. The title of this book is about teaching you new ways to eat and enjoy what you eat. Your brightest future will come from how you feel physically and mentally. Both things can be changed with a new lifestyle that no longer focuses on the salad you eat or the walk you took out of the mailbox.

Here are a few promises I will proclaim to you right now providing that you are coachable. To be coachable you must be open to new ideas and be ready to act on them. Enough of that since we both know you picked up this book because you are ready for the change to happen. Here are my guarantees:

1. You will feel better than ever if you stop stressing about food, exercise or anything else in your life.

2. You will lose the weight that you desire if you change your perspective on food and getting movement.

3. You will lose weight if you use your mind more in a constructive way.

4. You will feel like you can do more in life if you eat foods that make you feel happier.

5. Your attitude will improve as soon as you start to think differently.

Along the way I will make more guarantees but for now this will get you started. I want you to feel more empowered and I want you to know that the only way I will make guarantees is if I know them to be factual. The claims I make in this book have come from many years of research, real results from others who have followed my plan and my own personal results. I have lost over 150 pounds and have kept off the weight now for over three years.

My magic is no magic at all. It is just not the normal fad dieting type of stuff. I look for ways to take complicated subjects and ideas and dissect them so they can be broken down into the simplest form. I love helping myself by being the guinea pig first. Then I am committed to writing books and publications to help others after I have worked out the bugs. This is how I serve others.

In retrospect I guess my magic is that I can see things differently than most people and I will follow through to make things happen when I discover a better way. My magic can be your magic too if you will see what I see. If you follow through like I follow through then you will have magic too.

Once you begin to do this you will understand why I make the guarantees I do. I am not a doctor, and I am not making any medical claims. Everything I offer to you is strictly my opinion.

What is a fact to me must be checked out by you, tried, and implemented before it becomes a fact to you. I am just a guy who has had a lot of success with what I am about to present to you but, ultimately it will be up to you to see it through and determine if they are facts or not. How hard has it been to lose weight and feel great? When was the last time you felt incredible? Do you know how to feel great again? Here is the secret to life:

- Eat How You Want to Feel.
- Love how you want to be loved.
- Move how you want to be moved.
- Speak how you want to be spoken to.
- Think like you want to be thought of.
- And laugh often.

I say all of this to make a point. All too often people say one thing and then do something completely opposite. Nothing holds truer than people who want to lose weight, feel great and find true love. So, don't you think the best thing to do is do what you want to do? Shouldn't you star to act on your thoughts? I believe the answer is yes because you have sought out this book and it is all about doing what your heart desires with health and wellness.

At the beginning of this introduction, I started out by saying STOP! Now I say to you..... Go! Let's go and be what you really want, get the weight off you desire and get clarity on your health and wellness. I want to warn you before we get into the book and that is; my program is strong with mental exercises and mental strength exercises. Weight loss is more mental than physical. Now let's go!

Chapter 1
A Different Way of Thinking

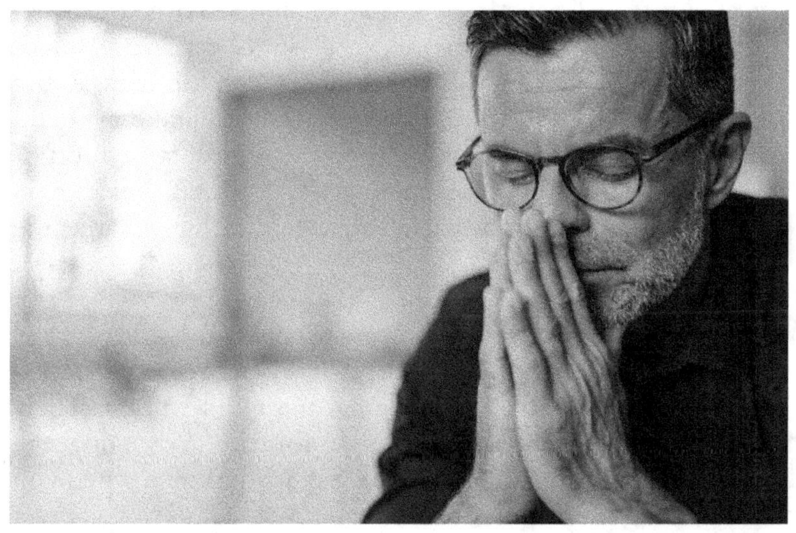

In 2013 I wrote the book How to Think Your Way to Thin. The main idea behind the book was how to lose weight using your mental powers. No, it is not voodoo or a weird book because your mind is very powerful and most of us are only using 8-10% of its capacity. Every percent you leverage in your frontal lobe does amazing things for you. That is as technical as I will get with you. Everything in that book is broken down as simply as I can lay it out. The book has changed so many lives and so now I wanted to add on to it with this book.

If you have not read the first book I would highly suggest that you grab a copy here. Either way this book will help you greatly, and although it is sequel of the other book (How To Think Your Way to Thin), it also can stand on its own.

This is a different way of thinking for most people, but the trend seems to be changing. Others have started to figure out what I have been saying all along. No matter what you do physically in this world, it all starts with your mind. The mind determines everything you do, and the trick is that you decide what your mind focuses on or it will take over and do it for you. When it comes to how you deal with food, if you move and get exercise and general overall health you want to be in charge because if you are not in charge the mind often protects you.

The protection that the mind often does for you is not always in your best interest. If you have had a bad experience or some kind of trauma, the mind will ultimately hold you back and not let you move forward. You know the kind of trauma I am talking about. Say for instance when you were dieting for instance in the past. Was it a great experience? Did you have a great time and lose all kinds of weight and feel healthier?

I bet if you are like most people it was not a great time and after a while of eating foods you didn't like and all that running turned out to be miserable. So, what your mind does is put up barriers to keep you from doing that again. It is a simple concept and makes sense to the mind. What doesn't make sense is how you get past these block walls and how you can go about weight loss and health in a different way.

What I am talking about is a different way of thinking. You need to start right now and change some thinking you may have. We need to remove barriers about your health, about losing weight and general overall happiness. Let me ask you a question; how often do you see someone who is healthy, in great shape and yet they are extremely miserable or a real downer? I bet you are thinking right now about people you know. I am not saying that it doesn't happen, but it is rare.

I will bring up happiness a lot throughout this journey you are on because it is important. Happiness is a state of mind along with weight loss and good health. There are many physical aspects you will have to partake in and follow through with but, here my pint and start with your thoughts. This is exactly how I have lost 150 pounds and have kept it off.

You can't fix everything with your mind but, you will be surprised how much you can affect in the way of change. I have found that the hardest part with my concept is that it is tough for people to think it is real. They struggle to believe that it is possible for them. "It seems like a mystical idea that is in another universe." Many have understood it and have been very successful but there are still so many that are apprehensive about giving it a try. The power of the mind is infinite, and it is up to each one of us to unlock it. This book is the beginning of unlocking that power.

Let's talk about three very important aspects of healthy living; losing weight, gaining energy and feeling great. Here is a fact; you are either gaining weight or losing weight all the time. It is so hard to stay at the same weight so if you do not want to gain weight then you will have to actively focus on small weight loss. I am talking no stress and weight loss. Lose a quarter pound a month but, whatever you do lose weight.

If you start to think differently then let's throw out the rules of typical dieting and weight loss. Be brave and bold and declare from here on out I will not stress about my weight or stress about weight loss or gain. You will not stress about what others think of you or how many times you have failed in the past. The stress game is a lose/lose game. Take a deep breath and let it out slowly. Okay now that you have washed away the stress we will talk about the no diet weight loss plan.

You will lose weight by doing some simple mental exercises and some physical exercises. The mental exercises will be explained in the next chapter. This will give you the actual mental exercises as well as some great physical exercises. I want to discuss more about why they will work for you.

The concept of why you can harness mental power is because your body listens to the mind. Everything you want to do is derived from the mind. The mind is also greatly under-utilized, and most people have no real clue what is possible. Sure, they have heard about only using 10% of the brain's capacity but, they really do not know what else is even possible. I am not a brain scientist, but I am a brain enthusiast.

As a brain enthusiast I have learned that so many things I thought I could not do before I now do with great ease. Some of it has come from experience and knowledge and some has come from maturity but, most has come from a deeper focus on what I want. I would bet if you were anything like me you do most things in your life by repetition and with little effort. Things like maybe reading a book, or driving, walking or maybe building widgets at work.

To leverage more from your mental capacity, you will have to hyper-focus in the areas you want to greatly change in. Areas like weight loss and health and wellness. You are doing your everyday routines, and you are getting along but, if you want to accelerate in these areas you will have to focus much deeper and train your mind what you want on a deeper more satisfying level.

When I was overweight by 150 pounds, my original focus was I don't care how much I weigh because I look good, and I am smart and charismatic and strong as an ox. One day that was no longer what I wanted so I changed my focus and said I wanted to lose weight, get healthy and wear smaller, better fitting clothes. Then I started to do something very important to start myself on the journey I had in mind; I started to vision what I wanted.

When most people want to lose weight they never usually have any goals in mind except maybe to fit into this or to not sweat so much when they play with their children. I had way deeper goals because if I achieved my goals then I would have all those basic benefits as an additional bonus.

I started having visions of what I looked like at every stage of my journey. I had specific pants sizes in my visions, shirt sizes and an overall look of my clothes and how they would fit. I also had visions that were in the present and not fantasies or if this happens

I might be like this. I had real conviction on my new body, and I also had convictions on my overall health and different aspects. Once I was concrete in my visions I went backwards to a point that I really wanted to change because weight gain is not often the result of eating too much. Weight gain is often the by-product of an unhealthy mind, choices and health issues.

For me it was a several fold problems (which is usually the case for everyone) that I needed to correct. I was type II diabetic and although it was relatively new for me I knew it was not a great thing to deal with. The medicines made me feel horrible and posed more problems than any good they were doing.

Next, I was doing really well for myself and owned a few businesses at the time. I was always eating on the go, at expensive restaurants where the meals were more of an event than a way to give me strength and energy. I drank too much (not excessive but excessive for healthy living) and I had not fully learned to manage my stress as I should have.

Lastly, my health and wellness were not a number one priority like it should have been. It was something I would deal with later but, guess what; it was now later and a huge priority. I didn't want to get to my forties, and they must do something about it. I heard so many stories over the years from forty somethings that talked about how hard it was to lose weight once they were forty plus. I now know that not to be the truth, but it turned out to be just the excuse I needed to change things around.

I went to work on getting my diabetes under control slowly getting myself off the medicine and keeping my sugar under control. I educated myself on what I needed to do to control my levels when it came to food and water and exercise.

After eight months I had accomplished my goals and visions. I still had not even lost any weight yet at this point. Pretty amazing considering I was over three hundred and fifty pounds or better. I always told people I was three hundred and thirty-six pounds because I was embarrassed at the weight I had hit, and I stopped checking my weight.

Next I went to work on choosing better foods, not eating on the run and totally changed why I ate. This brings me to a great point I want to bring up to you and really a few points I need to make at this point. Let me first start by asking you a thought-provoking question. Why do you eat food every day? What is your answer? If you are like me in any way I used to eat for comfort, because I was starving, to be social and because I could.

Why should you eat food? Your answer may be different than mine but, I suggest you consider my answer. I believe you should eat food to give your body the nutrients it needs. Take the social aspect out of it and the comfort and because you are starving. If you have the wrong focus with food it will come back to haunt you.

I started to eat to take care of my body's needs and for no other reasons. Here are some fast, hard rules to live by from here on out:

- Never have the feeling of being starved – EVER!
- Instead of eating 3 times a day – cat 6-9 times a day.
- Never feel bloated by overeating.
- When you need comfort because of a stressful situation, take comfort with a new activity like reading or golfing or gardening.
- Eat what makes you happy but, never eat too much of it at any given time.

These are some great rules that have shaped my new lifestyle and my plummet of one hundred and fifty pounds of weight loss and much better health. This is just the beginning of it all but a great place to start.

By now I am hoping you are getting a great sense of how far I have gone to change my health. I created visions, I created guidelines for eating and I began to really laser my focus on what I desired. I tapped into more of my mental capacity and made a true commitment to what was going to make happen in my life.

Your brain is no different than mine is (unless you have a medical issue with your brain that is) when it comes to what I have achieved and continue to achieve. You are underutilizing your mental capacity, and you can leverage it way more. This is not magic, but I have a different way of thinking, and as we continue with your journey it is important that you realize how seriously you must take all of this.

To better leverage your mental capacity, you will have to do mental exercises as well as physical ones. Have no fear though because I promise you that if I can do all of this, so can you.

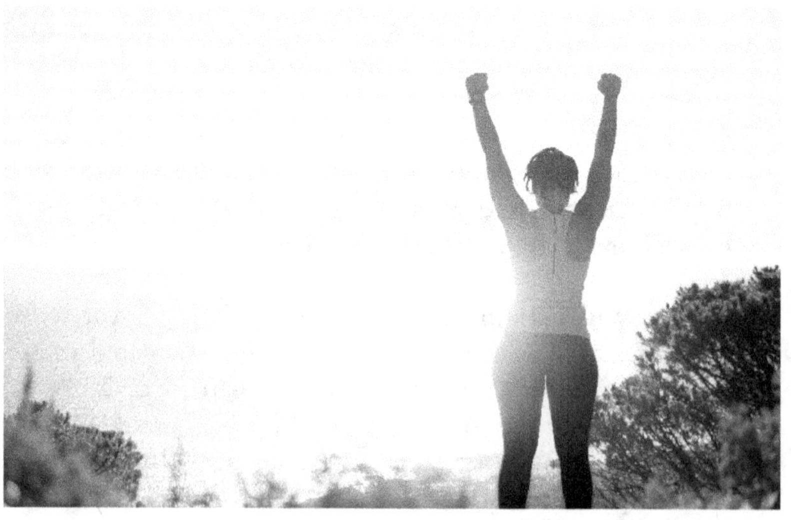

Chapter 2
Harnessing the Mind and Body

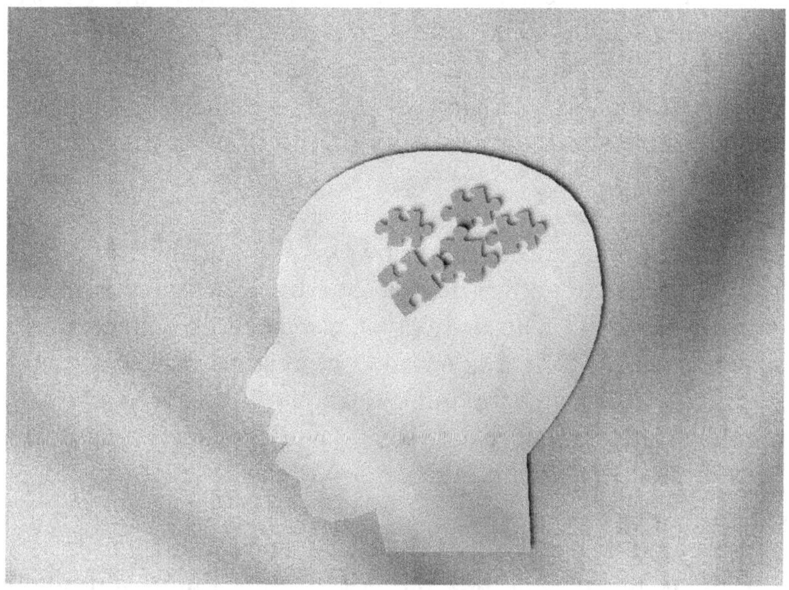

In chapter two we are going to learn about some of my mental exercises as well as some physical exercises. The first thing I would like to do is make a statement that may seem very elementary but must be stated clearly. The body will not operate at its peak without properly programming the mind. Sounds like a statement that I shouldn't have to state right? The truth is that I must state it and I need you to really understand it.

This book is not written for me per say. I write because of the joy and the motivation it brings me in helping people. Who the book is written for is you and because of that it is extremely important that it is you who understands every part of this program.

So, when I say that your mind and body must work together to achieve greatness, peace, a higher level or a pure healthy status then I pray you are clear on this statement and fact. Do not waste one minute fighting this idea because you will miss out on 70% of what this book is all about.

The big question is how do we get the mind and body to work together so we can harness the maximum capacity in you? The answer is; we need to set the mind straight and eat to feel good and get in some movement and re-enforce it all with the mind throughout. Let's look at my mental strategies and exercises so you can start to work on your mental strengthening.

One of the things I do every day when I get up is I am thankful for another day of health, mind and good fortune before my feet ever hit the ground. This is extremely important because how you start the day will be how you end the day. Never skip this activity.

The next exercise you need to do is remind yourself that food is fuel and every time you eat or drink something you are supercharging your machine. I visualize this all day long. Food is not my enemy as it is my rocket fuel. I create visions of a monster machine in my body and when I eat or drink it goes through the process of what it takes to rev up my machine to full capacity. You must create your own vision of what this looks like and then concentrate on it.

You must remember back to when your body was the best it was ever. A time when your weight was ideal, and you felt the very best. When you don't smoke, eat horrible fast food, or are out of breath when you take a short walk. Once you have a clear vision of this then you must focus on this new vision. This will be your new vision of who you are and never let it go. This becomes your new target and I do not care how impossible you think it is. This must be what you see in your mind as clearly as day.

As you are beginning to see in this program I created, it is very heavy with visual mind exercises for one reason; because they work. They work if you allow them and they work if you will do them. Visions are how the mind sees things as it remembers less about the words than it does the visions that it stores. Create the pictures in your mind that you want to create in your life.

Before we get into the foods, supplements and liquids we should taking in to feel how we want to start feeling, you will notice we have started with some exercises both mental and physical for one main reason; you need to get right before any food, or supplements are going to make a big impact.

At this point I also want you to forget about what you think you know about food or exercise. Let's start new information on what the possibilities are for a body who will treat itself better. You have incredible power inside of you. My job is to help you to realize it.

Mental exercises are as powerful if not more powerful as physical exercises. Take the time necessary to build your mental muscles just as you would your biceps, triceps and any other muscles in your body. By doing this you will help make any physical exercise more powerful and impactful.

Building your mental muscles starts with spending more time alone and with your thoughts building your self-esteem, visions, cleansing yourself of any impure thoughts that are self-destructing to your desired reality. By practicing this you will return yourself to a thinner, healthier and happier human being which is what you were meant to be.

One of my favorite things to do every day is to visualize physical exercises in my mind while I do low impact physical exercises. For instance, if I am visualizing sit ups then I will at the same time work on contracting and tightening my stomach muscles. There are many types of similar exercises that can be done like this and no matter where you are with your health you can do these.

The bottom line to harnessing your mind is to clear it of all doubt and clutter focus more on what you want and exercise it several times a day.

Chapter 3
Start a Garden and Grow Your Own Food

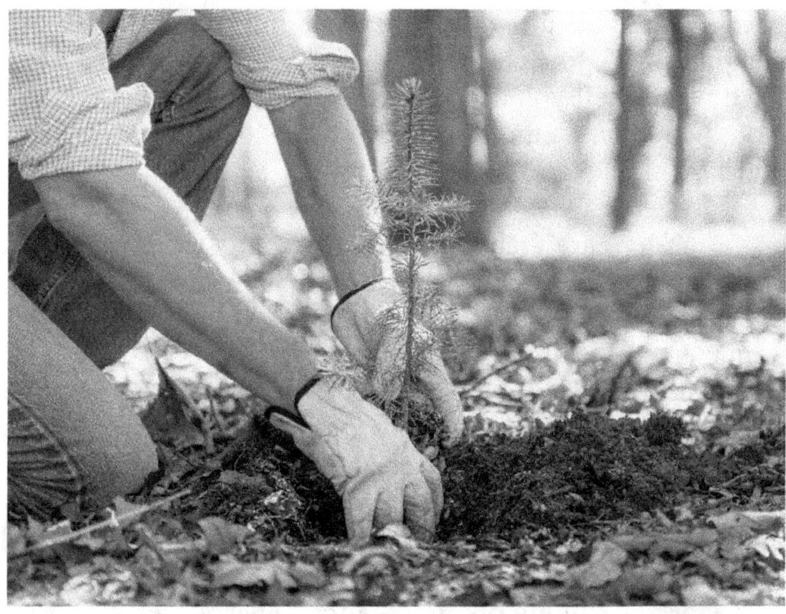

I am certain that your schedule is already full and many of you may even barely have time to stop and take a nap every blue moon but, what good is being busy if you are living unhealthily.

When I have conversations with people who want to lose weight they are always telling me how they are too busy and when I make suggestions about how to change their health, most people make sounds of exhaustion and claim they are so busy. I am not trying to contradict them but that idea of being too busy is what is building more fast-food restaurants, quick grab and go junk food and more coffee houses.

Time is an illusion and how much time you have is relevant to how you allocate that time. Better stated is you have all the time that you need it is just a matter of how you are spending it. If you consider that idea even for a second then you can begin on the path to regaining your health and happiness. If you consider what I am saying about time then when I tell you that starting a garden is a good idea for you then the next thing out of your mouth will not be that I have no time.

There are many reasons why I am stating you must start your own garden and we will look at every one of those reasons but, first we also need to understand a few things about healthy eating. The first thing is that we have followed a food chart most of our lives. You know the chart I am talking about as it is the same one that started for you in kindergarten. The food chain or chart that shows how much bread you should eat, amount of protein and how much milk to drink. Have you ever studied the chart, and do you understand if what they have taught you is even right for you? In my opinion the food chart is not a one size fits all way for everyone to eat and the chart is flawed. Every single person is different and what they need in the way of nutrition is different in every case.

I will not get too deep into the food chart and why it is flawed but I will try my best to make something clear in the hopes that I can motivate you to investigate it some more. The chart is flawed, wrong and what is recommended for you is not right. So do yourself a big favor and search the food chart in Google and see what you can discover.

Then I want you to try and go a week and eat like it recommends to you and discover how you feel. What I know and suspect is that you will not feel great and if you keep it up for too long then you will also probably put on some weight gain as well.

Speaking of food and what is in it, let's talk about food labels. Do you even have a clue what is in the food that you are picking up off the shelf at the grocery store? Are they in alignment with the food chart recommended by the U.S.D.A.? My biggest grip of everything I talk about is that there are 50 plus different names for sugar and most people only know about four of them off the top of their head.

Sugar is the enemy so make no mistake about it. Sugar is the new drug of choice for Americans, and I suspect of other countries as well. Sugar is addicting and so much, so it is being put into so many things that you buy from the grocery store.

Recently from a documentary I saw on television about sugar, they stated that even tomato paste is full of sugar. Why do you need sugar in tomato paste? Outrageous to think you are getting tomatoes and other herbs and not to realize they have laced it with sugar.

Besides the ugly side effects, sugar is addicting to the mind and body. Just watch someone who was an alcoholic once. I would suspect they crave sugar in the form of cookies, ice crème, candy and more. That beer belly we are all too familiar with is more of a sugar belly. Alcohol is full of sugar, and it tends to go straight to the belly.

If I haven't started to convince you just yet that it might be time to start growing your own food and a garden then maybe a few more things might. Did you know that certain fast-food restaurants wash their beef with some nasty chemicals that would not be fit even for a pig? Also, ground beef is also washed in a similar chemical that supposedly makes it edible for consumption.

Before you vegans and vegetarians get too excited, natural sources of vitamin b come from meat and poultry. We need this source but, why is there no better way to treat beef? Also, why can't food labels use language that is plain, clear and understandable? If we are trying to supposedly help people make healthy decisions then why can't the food industry seem to get these labels right?

I am not trying to put down the food industry but, the consumer needs to understand that the labels and marketing for foods are by design. Like cigarette companies of the past, food companies want to get you hooked on their products and keep you hooked. They do not care if you have diabetes or an irritable bowl or Crohn's disease.

They only care about profits. Social responsibility to them is donating a check to save the local animal shelter. They do not seem fazed by the fact they are poisoning the people in this country and others. As a company or industry, they should focus on profits but, when the pursuit of profits is continually taking down one person after another with afflictions then profits should no longer be the goal at hand.

Big business and government push us as far as they can before they finally back off. The food industry goes about things in a little different way but, still push none the less. If we make enough people aware of what is really going on than we can start to change people's lives. This book is about realizing what makes your body feel the best. Too much of anything will tear it down and cause health issues. Even water will kill you if you have way too much at one sitting.

What exactly is in that box of Mac and Cheese, Oreos, or cupcakes is hard to explain. The ingredients are mostly not very quality in nature but, they are cheap to produce for the companies producing them. There are exceptions available and there are plenty of alternatives but sadly you really must watch what you put in your basket or pick up in that drive through the window.

I know growing your own fruits and vegetables is not the entire answer but, then again, there is never going to be a one size answer to fix everything. Solid change is continual, small incremental change. Start with taking some of the toxins out of your diet and replacing them with better choices. Every little change of habit adds up.

Chapter 4
Feel Good Foods Your Body Will Crave

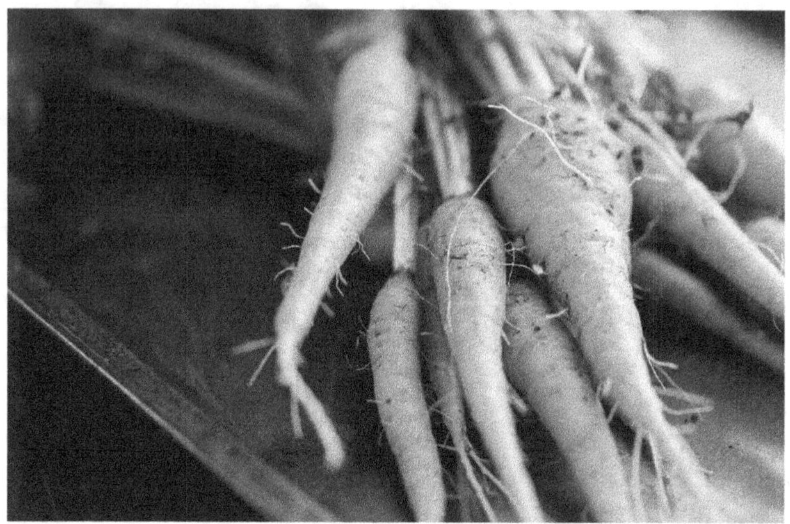

If you eat so that you can fuel your body and feel great, what is the best case for you when it comes to eating? How do you want to feel every time you are done eating? Let me pose a thought for you and then maybe we can work on this problem of food and eating and help move you forward.

If we went back not too many years ago, most people would have to go out and hunt their food and grow their food. Some people might say to that statement thank goodness. Thank God technology has advanced and it easy to go to the grocery store and buy a basket full of food. The problem is that the food in the grocery store is not that healthy, and you buy everything cheap you can get your hands on. I am not passing judgment towards you because it is the way things are and in today's times we can no longer just live off the land.

We have already discussed the problem with our food today but in this case it is the physical aspects of what we used to do for our food. We were active and yet today we do so little compared to just 100 years ago. In fact, we are even less active than just 30 years ago. If we can no longer hunt our own foods then what can we do? My answer is twofold; one is to get active and two is to eat foods that are a real source of energy and give you that great feeling.

Let's set some hard and fast rules for eating and then we can suggest some foods that can boost your mood and health. If you can set these ideas straight in your mind ahead of time then you will set a great foundation before we even get too specific on the types of foods to eat.

The first rule is that we will no longer sit down and pound too much food into our belly at anyone sitting and in fact you agree to wait 90 minutes in between eating any food. Once you walk away from what you are eating you will not go back for more in less than 90 minutes in between.

When I was 150 pounds overweight I started with this rule first. I would stop sitting down to a meal and eat until it hurt, had bloating or that terrible lethargic feeling. I knew that once I felt like any of these ways that I was done with. To put this into perspective take your fist and lift it up and stare at it. This is how big your stomach is before eating food. Now, look at all the food on your plate at dinnertime. Are you starting to see the problem?

Since I was always over stretching my stomach I did not want to exercise, walk or work or do anything for that fact. Do you relate to what I am saying? Have you also had these problems too? So, let's agree that from this day forward you will no longer cause yourself any more harm by over stuffing your stomach.

If you are no longer going to overeat at anyone sitting then how do you get the right amount of food in your stomach that your body craves? That brings us to the second rule and that is to eat small meals or snacks all day long and in fact every 90 minutes to 120 minutes. Why does this make sense to do? The answer is simple; not only does it accomplish our first rule but, your body will begin to thank you for the massive energy that it will receive. Constantly eating all day in small bites gives your body a source of renewed energy.

The next rule you need to agree to is that food is no longer thought of with a guilty mind. Eat healthy choices with the goal in mind of increasing your metabolism and feeling great.

Now that we have a few rules established let's talk about, focus on and analyze feel-good foods. My definition of feel-good foods are foods that energize you, do not make you feel bad and that you enjoy eating. Let's face it; if you are not excited about what you are eating then you will never have control over your weight.

Many times, throughout my life I tried to eat salads and nuts and berries so to speak and I was miserable. It was not because I do not like salads or berries but because if was restricted to only these types of foods then I felt trapped. Freedom in anything is empowering. I do not necessarily want the freedom to eat crappy and unhealthy food although we all love a cupcake or candy bar from time to time. Freedom to enjoy the food we desire is enjoyable and will make you the happiest.

I do often choose those foods that I know will provide my body with the fuel that it desires but foods that taste great and that I enjoy also need to be an option. My point is that you need to always be happiest to live healthily.

Chapter 5
Natural Solutions to Fuel Your Body

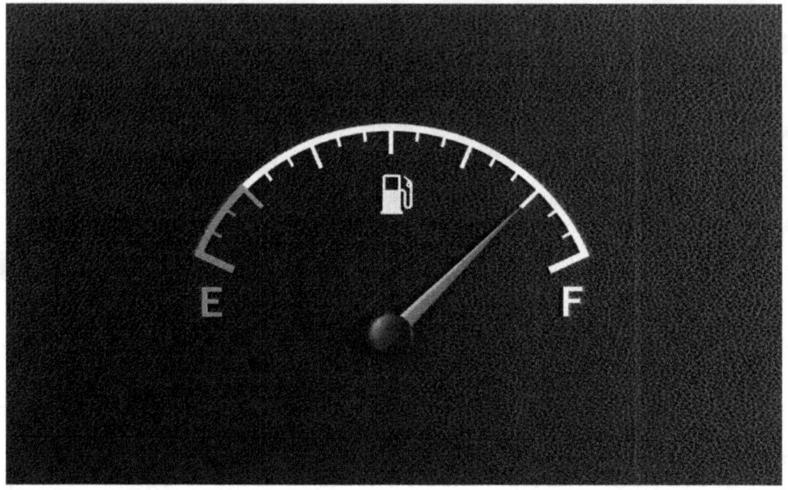

To get started we need to make sure that you properly hydrate. Too little water in your diet will cause you lots of problems both short term and long term. It is not about gulping down water at one sitting but, constantly giving your body the water it needs and craves.

Your skin will look healthier and more youthful, you will stay regular and flush your body of bad waste and weight loss will become easier. I caution you that drinking too much water at one time can harm you so make sure you do your homework. If you are like most people you are not drinking nearly enough water.

I am not a big fan of medicines or drugs. They have their place and uses, and if you need them then take them of course. For me I try and put natural solutions in my body as often as possible. A good multivitamin, aloe vera, vitamin B's, vitamin C, magnesium and more is what your body can prosper from. Everything we need to live healthily is grown naturally here on earth and not necessarily manufactured in a lab.

There are many stories out there and more coming about every day about the power of naturopathic medicines or remedies. A special root that helps with arthritis or a berry mix that cures cancer. Natural anti-oxidants or natural energy or metabolism boost all are here for your body if you will seek them out. They are not voodoo or a waste of time or money. Natural remedies are what are best for your body. Foreign things going into your body cause long term effects. We live in a perfect world for optimal health and wellness but, it has become unpopular to do the hard work needed to extract these properties or pay for them as they can be expensive.

A great question to ask here though is how expensive is unhealthy living? How expensive are medications, health care and lost time at work or your business? The answers are they are exponentially more expensive than these vitamins, minders and supplements. Make some alterations to your budget and fit them in.

In my opinion, the methods I use are to research natural solutions that help me with things that are good for my body or any issue I may be having. Then I research to figure out how much of a dose is effective for what I need. Then I try them and monitor my health and adjust as I go.

I communicate with my doctor as often as possible to alert her as to the fact I am taking them to make sure they do not interfere with treatment. d to determine if there is any harm to me for some unknown reason. To date I have not had any conflicts, but it is always wise to work with your doctor regarding your health.

Let's take a moment to talk about doctors, medication and the for-profit health care system out there. Your doctor is probably smart as far as things go. Any person who sacrifices over eight years of their life and gets a medical degree deserves respect. With, give them respect for their accomplishment and move on. You are your best doctor at the end of the day. I make this statement even though you have no degree from a prestigious university and do not get the paycheck to go with it. Your doctor has a minimum of eight years but, if you are 40 years old then you should have 40 years' worth of education about your body. No two bodies are the same and yours is unique to only you. Be a student and learn about your body and what ails it and what it will take to be your healthiest.

Some of the supplements I also suggest looking into are Mega3, flaxseed, chia seed, Alpha lipoic acid, L acetyl carnitine, L cystine, Co enzyme Q10, lecithin – no GMO and all the B vitamins. These supplements are great for inflammation and nerve repair. They help with several ailments and help to lead to good health.

You should also Find a water filter that removes acidity and neutralizes the water. Another great source of illness in your body is drinking acidic water and acidic drinks. It can be expensive but, again, so is bad health.

Natural supplements, herbs and natural healing take a lot of research and long-term commitment on your part. Do not look for miracles overnight. Stay fast and feed your body all this goodness. Finding the right doses for your body is important.

Price is important to you I am sure as there is so much goodness your body needs. Do your research. I do not buy all my supplements from the same place although I buy a lot from Amazon and quite a bit from GNC. Do your homework and make your budget work. I am sure you are spending money on poison for your body now in some way or another so remove some poison and replace it with healthy supplements.

Lastly, let's not forget good old fruits and vegetables, roots, and herbs that are right here on earth as well. My personal favorite is to juice as much as I can. It is a bit time-consuming but well worth it.

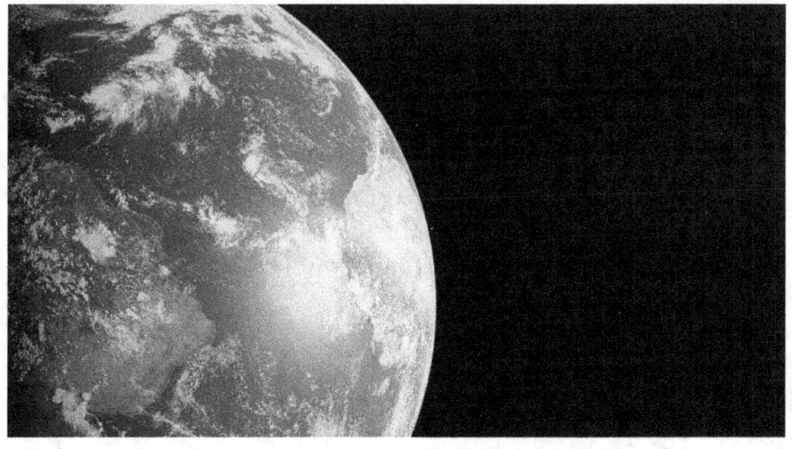

Chapter 6
Listen and Learn From Your Body

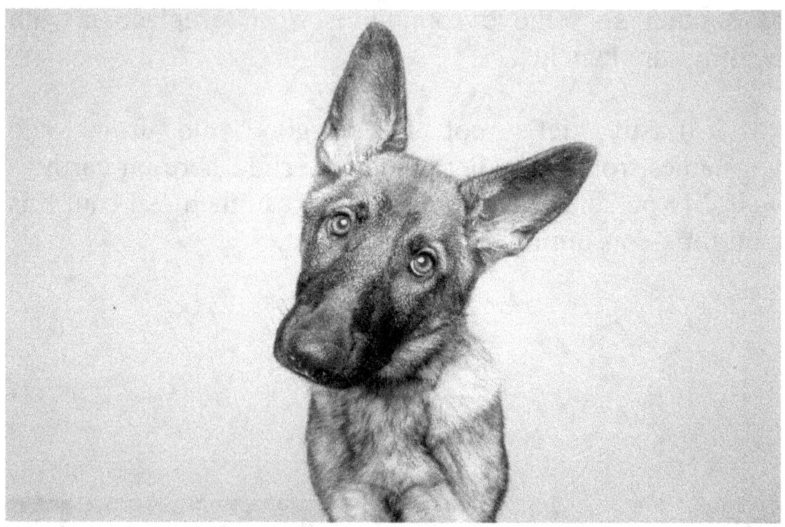

I believe the number one rule in health and wellness and weight loss is to listen to your body. You must be willing to pay attention to the good and bad of what your body is trying to tell you. If you fail to listen to the warning signs then you will surely pay the price. Let me tell you a story about how I did not listen to my body.

It had been several years since I had been working on my feet doing hard labor. I had been a contractor and did remodel work and could work seven days a week and 10 plus hours a day but, then again, I was younger. Fast forward six years later after being off my feet like that I took on a major remodel job. I worked those seven days a week and ten hours a day schedule I described above once again. I lasted about three weeks, and I formed a blister on my big toe and seven months later I was still not healed and had an infection in a second toe.

Now if I had started with common sense I would have thought better than to go charging right back into something so intense. Secondly, I had many signs leading up to this injury and if I paid attention to my body I would never have had to endure the pain and agony I went through.

To start with my feet started to ace almost right away. I don't mean just feeling tired but ached. Next I started to feel like I had a horrible case of shin splints. Then I had a small blister that formed, and the wound hurt me bad. I was sick feeling and my feet felt like they weighed three hundred pounds. If I was better at listening to my body like I normally do I would have heard the cry for relief and care. No onc clse knows your body better than you do and no one else can hear your bodies cry better than you can.

Your body is brilliantly designed to communicate with you. It will tell you when you are hungry, if you have eaten too much and if it is tired. Your body will tell you if it is hurt, sick or bent out of shape. You will know if you are feeling young, old or feeling your age. You have a great communication system in you if you are willing to listen to it and act on its requests.

If you are feeling under the weather lately or are lacking the energy you desire or need to lose weight then the key to better health is in you. Be a student of your body and take notes so you end up in a better place.

Chapter 7
Move with a Purpose

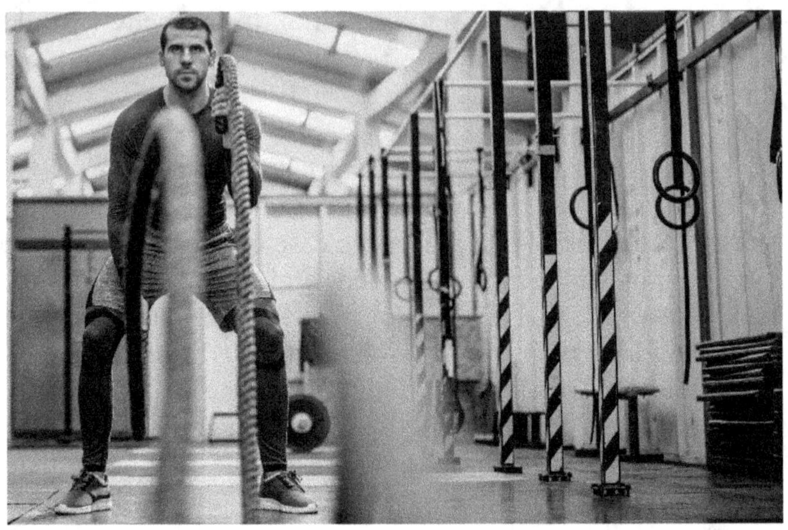

I know you may not like to hear this but, a body in motion tends to stay in motion. Yes that means we need to get you moving to whatever degree you can move. You need to get back to that state when you were young and free and full of energy. You will have to determine what your limitations are, but I urge you to get your mind and your body moving and only stop when you need rest.

I am aware that you may have limitations right now, and then to have some strangers tell you that you need to get moving while you start some sort of exercise is probably not what you were looking for when you bought this book.

Honestly, good health does not come from rest as much as it does from movement. Your body was meant to move, stretch, resist, elongate, and when you sit around too much you are putting too much pressure on your body and stiffening up your joints. The more you sit, the more you will become lethargic. The less you move the less you will be able to move. The more lethargic you become the less you will want to move as the day moves on.

Even if you are bound in a wheelchair you still can get moving. I know because I am in one and I move a ton in my daily life. This will hold true unless you are completely disabled. Remember to always ask your doctor what you can do with respect to exercise. If you can move parts of your body then you should get moving those parts including your mind.

Do you want to know the heaviest object in this world? The heaviest object in this world is stress, and the pressure it creates on your body is both good as well as bad stress. How can you get moving if you are bearing that weight? It is not enough to make statements about removing stress in your life. Your doctor can say it until he or she is blue in the face but, until a new reality comes over you the words will never matter.

What is stress? Do not get nervous as I am no scientist or doctor or a stress expert and in fact all I really am a student of what I want in life. I have no technical jargon and in fact my real specialty is taking things that are complicated in nature and I break them down to the simplest form for others to understand better. In this case I want to help you to better understand stress, what part you are allowing it to play and how you can combat the effects that it is having on your life and body.

The way I think about stress I have the good stress that can create the kind of pressure that gets me moving. We all need a nudge from time to time and good stress can do that for me. Good stress or what I really like calling it is the motivator. The motivator puts the right amount of pressure and urgency te motivator is that extra fuel you need to peak in your performance. There are no side effects and there is no weight gain or fatigue. The motivator will supply you with the energy necessary to get the job done no matter what it may be.

Sources of good stress come from having goals and dreams where you finally decide to accomplish something great. When you decide to finally grab your dreams or even complete something small but significant then you apply the amount of pressure you need to get moving.

This comes in the form of deadlines you demand of yourself or maybe even a benchmark like the first ten pounds of weight to drop. The pressure comes from how your new pants size will feel or the amounts of money you will have in your bank account. The motivation is just what the doctor ordered for health and prosperity or that is my philosophy at least.

So, for every good in this world there is the opposite side of things and in this case that is bad stress. Bad stress or the five-thousand-pound gorilla sitting on your shoulders is the weight that is suffocating your chest. It is stealing life right out from you and is keeping you frozen.

Stress is where that extra weight is coming from around your belly and is what is always making you tired every day. The gorilla is big and tough and mean and wants to make you feel the weight and the pressure you are burdening. This pressure makes you want to give up and lie down and not get up and get moving.

The Gorilla gets its beginnings from pressure put on by others and situations not in your control. This is the perfect vehicle for the gorilla to jump on our shoulders and get busy breaking you down and slowing you down. There really is nothing good about the gorilla except for one thing; the gorilla is only real if you allow him to be real. The gorilla will only weight you down if you allow him a place in your life. When you decide that the gorilla has no place in your life and that you are kicking him out, then you will finally be ready to live a happier existence.

You are in control in all situations even when bad things happen to you. I am not saying bad things are your fault but, what you have control over is how you react, feel and move when it occurs. Even as I made that statement some of you started to get heated over what I wrote. That is the gorilla wanting to move right back in your life. Stop it from happening before things get out of control.

There are many techniques to work on removing stress and everyone is different in what works for them. Stress is a tricky subject and I hate to tell you exactly what I feel for fear that some of you are so stressed you might take offense. The truth is though if you knew me you would know I tell it like it is. You see this is a way I avoid stress in my life. I just say it like it is because it is healthier for me and for the receiver even if they do not think so.

The truth about stress is that you can decide how things make you feel and then decide how you are going to deal with it. I am probably just as guilty as you are when I say that people stress me out. The truth is I was the one that stressed myself out based upon how I felt about someone else. Their behavior may not be that great or they did something wrong but let's be truthful as you get to decide what it means to you.

I know it is not easy to just say you should not let it bother you but, what if you could do this with half of these issues? You could wipe away half of your stress just by deciding that you will not react to certain people like you have. The words I said are you get to decide and because of this you have control. The rest of the situations are probably harder and need to work hard on dealing with them.

In the meantime, you can wipe away the first fifty percent with little effort I promise you. The feelings that get attached to people or situations that stress you out are all determined by you. No one is forcing you to feel a certain way.

If you disagree with anything I am saying then I challenge you to explain what stress is and how it happens to you. If you put stress in the hands of anyone else or some mystical object then what you are saying is that it is out of your control and that my friend would stress me out.

I am certain by now you agree with me that how you deal with stress is up to you and because of that you should feel empowered to finally get your health and life under control. Once the stress starts to melt away then you can start to really get moving and feel alive. You will want to get moving more as soon as you remove the gorilla from your life.

Chapter 8
Why Dieting Fails Most of the Time?

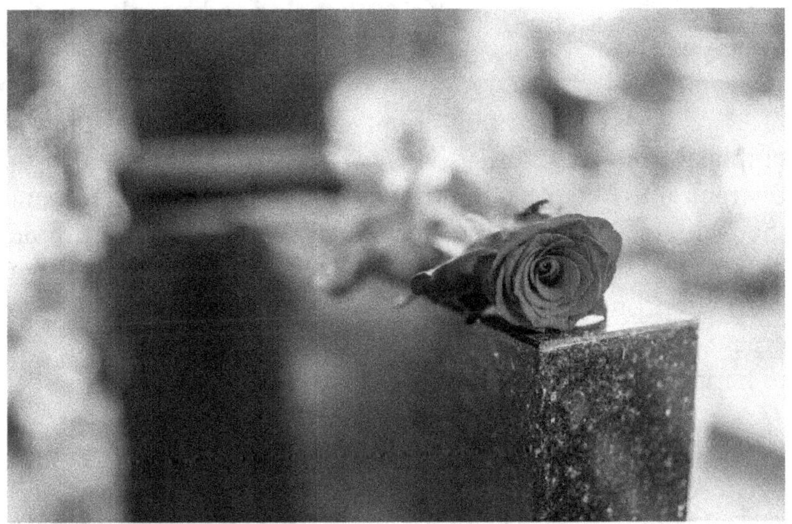

Have you ever wondered why most people fail on "die"ts? An even better question might be how do some people have success with a diet plan while others fail miserably? I mean if a thousand people go on a diet maybe one or two will lose the amount of weight they desire and keep it off. Do you think this is because they were on a special diet plan through one of those national diet companies? Maybe they are just lucky or did things only they could do. Maybe they have money and people who have money can lose weight any time they want, right?

If you have read my first book called "How to Think Your Way to Thin," then you already know that none of that is true. Rule number one is that everyone can lose weight once they decide that is what they want and have a desire to be healthier and skinnier than where you currently are. If you have read my other book The Lies We Tell Ourselves then you also know that excuses and lies have no part in your life. You must always be real in order to be your best.

The simple truths about diets are that they put an emphasis on the word "DIE." The T is simply there to distract you. When you and your body get out of alignment then a correction is needed. This should be a simple correction and some mental exercises along with a correction on how you eat and what you are doing. If we create a situation where we feel deprived or where we get unhappy then weigh loss is less likely

Successful diet programs or plans do work at times because they have a system for people to follow and structure in how to do something is very important for most people to be a part of. Next they generally provide a support system for their clients which is very important for the success of almost anything in life.

The most important ingredient for a successful diet program is to get the participants to buy into it 100% and not question the journey they are on and follow everything laid out for them to a tee. The problem with this is that people never follow anything that is exact and even worse is that they then feel dependent on the system in order not to put the weight back on. Long term this is a recipe for disaster. People need to know that they can do it with the program or on their own.

My methods are different, but they are effective. My methods work because they help people just like you to realize the keys to their success are already inside them. People just often need a reminder from time to time from someone on the outside looking in. I am not emotional about how you feel or the weight you have put on. I am a cheerleader for you to help you awaken and be who you want. I am your mental trainer who will help set your mind straight again and show you the way.

What you need to succeed with your weight loss goals or healthier lifestyle is to know that you can make anything you want to happen as long as you are focused. If you let doubt creep in then you will surely suffer setbacks.

Chapter 9
Find the Support You Need in Order to Succeed

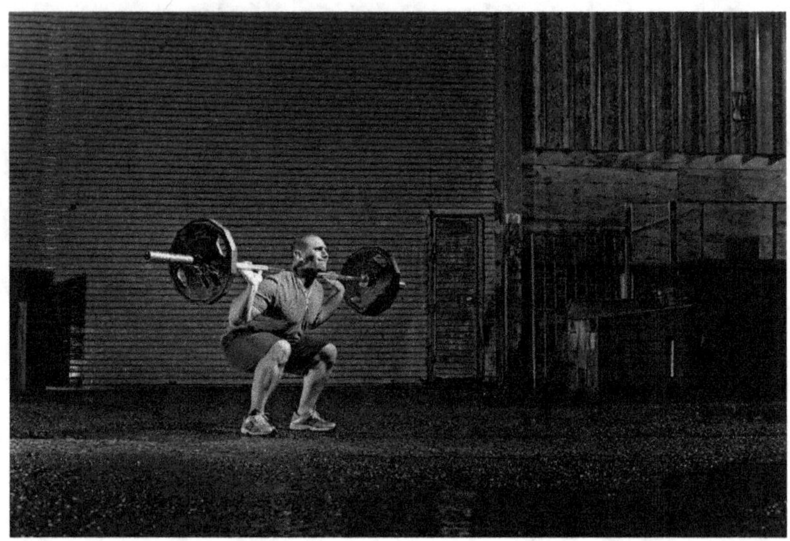

The success and dynamics of a group are determined by how well the group works together to support and lift the others up in the group. When a group of people work as a team or a cohesive unit then the magic that occurs is wonderful to witness. We have needs of support and great leadership as human beings. Support helps us to stay focused, on track and accountable for what we really want and that is why you should see out a support system to help you succeed as well.

I am not talking about a workout partner or a group of partners. If you need that then by all means do that as well. What I am talking about is finding others who support a healthier lifestyle and help each other with things like recipes, growing food together, searching information on alternatives, and other aspects.

Moral support is very important especially if you have not been eating healthily or exercising or doing any of the activities described in this book. The fact is we all get weak at times and need someone on the team to lift us up. You are not a weak person because you seek help after all even a Hall of Fame Pitcher throws a horrible game from time to time and needs moral support from his teammates.

I started my company Truth Mastery because I understood in those early days that most people need a deeper level of support. I wanted my company to be a part of the solution for people and not the problem. We help by coaching people daily to stay accountable for what they really desire.

Chapter 10
Where Do You Go From Here?

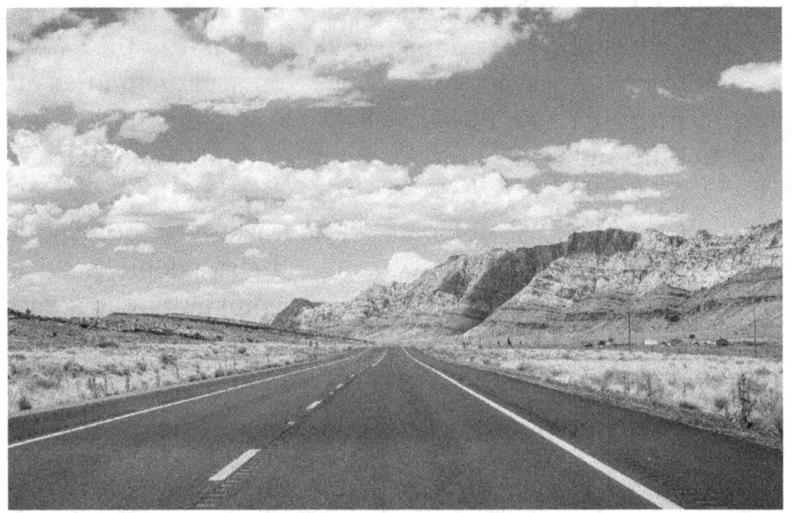

The journey you can embark on from here can be not only very rewarding but can be exciting every day. I tend to have fun with everything I do, and when I embark on a new adventure such as this I like to make it a game. I like to see how far I can make it or how much better I feel each day about what I am doing. Eating healthy and living healthy has many rewards to it. Do not look at this as something you "have" to do. Look at this as something you want to do because you deserve to feel your best.

When I started on my journey to losing over 140 pounds I was not really   excited at first, but I knew that losing weight was not the goal. I knew living a healthier life would bring me great joy, let me do more without being tired or sweating. I knew my clothes would it better and I would feel better about myself. The journey I was embarking on far outweighed what I felt that I was giving up. Once I got started I had a whole new perspective on what I should be doing.

Eat how you want to feel is a title I felt that would convey a clear meaning for what you should be doing with your body and life. I wanted to paint a clear picture for you to begin to understand what your possibilities are for your future.

I know it has gotten tougher to find better alternatives to eating but a great place to start is to drive past the drive-through of those fast-food places you once frequented. Carry around a cooler in your car if you must for when you get hungry and in fact as I stated earlier eat often in small feedings. This is a big secret to healthier living and weight loss and even if you do not follow the rest of the book this alone will do wonders for you.

So, there you have it for this phase of our new lifestyle. I encourage you to pick up my other books on Amazon and I would love to hear your thoughts on this book via a review.

It has been my pleasure serving you and I believe I have delivered value and enrichment to you and your life. I would love to hear our success stories as you get started and progress through your journey. You can connect with me at Robert@truthmastery.com

I wish you nothing but the best and I believe in you and hope you do too!

Chapter 11
About the Author Robert Kintigh

I know my best days are always ahead of me and I pray the same holds true for you.

I began my writing career with the hopes of reaching out to as many human beings as possible, and I wat to touch their lives in a special way. My writing style has always been to give the simple truth of things without all the jargon and scientific verbiage. The human brain is very complex and so is the body but as people we are simple, and we need it in whatever plain language that we speak.

When I write I try and do the following:
- I always try to be honest in my words and assessment.
- I will try to speak to you and not at you.
- I try and take complicated subjects and make them so any level of intelligence can understand it.
- I try and be 100% real and me.
- I go to work every day learning new things and discovering new truths to share with my audience.
- I try to speak from the heart and let my mind take a second seat.
- Lastly, I believe that we are an incredible species and even though we fail a lot we have incredible potential not yet realized.

Robert has degrees in business and leadership amongst other subjects, but his first love is writing. A thirst for being that voice that tells things in a way that you can relate to and not shy away from. He loves helping others and mentoring as many people as is possible. He does not believe in handouts but loves to give a hand up.

Raised in a town in southern California by the name of Downey California, he now lives and resides in Boise, Idaho. This environment allows him to feel creative, one with nature and a love for the simpler time in life.

Robert's company is Truth Mastery and is named after his first book called The Lies We Tell Ourselves where Robert helps you to eliminate your lies, discover your truths, and design your success. You discover how to live your truths!

If you are looking for a speaker for your next event, if you need a coach or a mentor then contact Robert today to see if the timing will work out for you. I promise you that it will be the best investment that you have ever made.

Robert has raised three children and now helps to raise many grandchildren to date. The next chapter in Robert's story is still being written but he has exciting things lined out for his future.

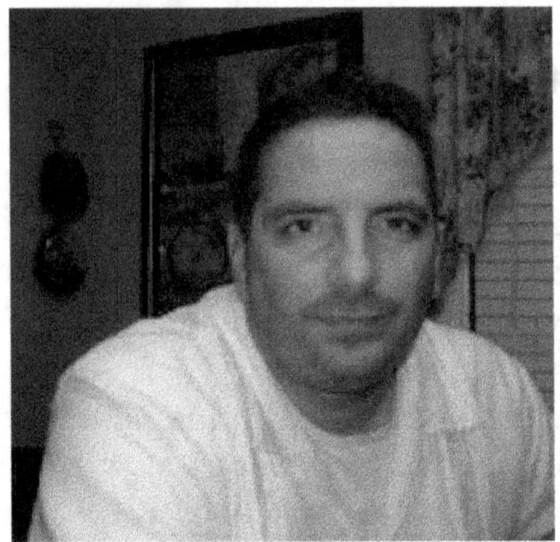

Figure 1 Picture Robert Kintigh

Figure 2 Copyright © Truth Mastery logo